Name: _____

Phone: _____

Email: _____

* * *

Doctor's name: _____

Phone: _____

Email: _____

* * *

**Emergency
contact:** _____

Phone: _____

Mobile: _____

CONTENTS

Blood Sugar Tables

> I can't change the direction of the wind, but I can adjust my sails to always reach my destination.
>
> JIMMY DEAN

Blood Sugar Targets

Time to Check	Standard Targets	My Targets	My Usual Results
Before meals	80-130 mg/dl	_____ to _____	_____ to _____
	4.5-7.3 mmol/l	_____ to _____	_____ to _____
Two hours after start of meals	Less than 180 mg/dl	Less than _____	Less than _____
	Less than 10 mmol/l	Less than _____	Less than _____
Bedtime	90-150 mg/dl	_____ to _____	_____ to _____
	5.0-8.3 mmol/l	_____ to _____	_____ to _____

Blood Sugar Levels

Type	Before Meal		After Meal (2 hours)
	Minimum	**Maximum**	
Normal	70 mg/dl	100 mg/dl	Less than 140 mg/dl
	4 mmol/l	6 mmol/l	Less than 7.8 mmol/l
Pre-diabetes	100 mg/dl	125 mg/dl	140-200 mg/dl
	6.1 mmol/l	6.9 mmol/l	7.8-11.1 mmol/l
Diabetes	More than 125 mg/dl	------------	More than 200 mg/dl
	More than 7 mmol/l	------------	More than 11.1 mmol/l

HbA1c Levels

Type	mmol/mol	%
Normal	Less than 42 mmol/mol	Less than 6.0%
Pre-diabetes	42-47 mmol/mol	6.0-6.4%
Diabetes	48 mmol/mol and up	6.5% and up

Blood Sugar to HbA1c Conversion

HbA1c (%)	HbA1c (mmol/mol)	Avg. Blood Glucose (mmol/L)
13	119 mmol/mol	18 mmol/L
12	108 mmol/mol	17 mmol/L
11	97 mmol/mol	15 mmol/L
10	86 mmol/mol	13 mmol/L
9	75 mmol/mol	12 mmol/L
8	64 mmol/mol	10 mmol/L
7	53 mmol/mol	8 mmol/L
6	42 mmol/mol	7 mmol/L
5	31 mmol/mol	5 mmol/L

Calorie Expenditure Guide

> **Only I can change my life,**
> **no one can do it for me.**
>
> CAROL BURNETT

Calorie Expenditure Guide

LIGHT PHYSICAL ACTIVITIES	IN 1 HOUR	IN 30 MIN
Sleeping	60	30
Watching TV	70	35
Sitting (reading)	100	50
Standing	110	55
Driving	110	55
Office Work	110	55

MODERATE PHYSICAL ACTIVITIES	IN 1 HOUR	IN 30 MIN
Cooking	220	110
Billiards	220	110
Bowling	260	130
Weight lifting	270	135
Volleyball	270	135
Auto repair	270	135
Walking	360	180
Hatha Yoga / Stretching	360	180
Gardening	400	200
Carpentry	400	200

VIGOROUS PHYSICAL ACTIVITIES		
Aerobic (low impact)	490	245
Skiing (downhill)	530	265
Jogging	530	265
Dancing (fast)	530	265
Rowing (stationary)	620	310
Tennis	620	310
Hockey	710	355
Basketball	710	355
Skiing (cross-country)	710	355
Bicycling	710	355
Running	800	400
Swimming	890	445

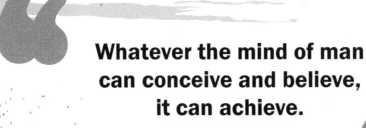

**Whatever the mind of man
can conceive and believe,
it can achieve.**

NAPOLEON HILL

Estimated Daily Calorie Needs

Estimated Daily Calorie Needs

Activity level	MALE		
Age (years)	Sedentary	Moderately active	Active
2	1,000	1,000	1,000
3	1,200	1,400	1,400
4	1,200	1,400	1,600
5	1,200	1,400	1,600
6	1,400	1,600	1,800
7	1,400	1,600	1,800
8	1,400	1,600	2,000
9	1,600	1,800	2,000
10	1,600	1,800	2,200
11	1,800	2,000	2,200
12	1,800	2,200	2,400
13	2,000	2,200	2,600
14	2,000	2,400	2,800
15	2,200	2,600	3,000
16	2,400	2,800	3,200
17	2,400	2,800	3,200
18	2,400	2,800	3,200
19 - 20	2,600	2,800	3,000
21 - 25	2,400	2,800	3,000
26 - 30	2,400	2,600	3,000
31 - 35	2,400	2,600	3,000
36 - 40	2,400	2,600	2,800
41 - 45	2,200	2,600	2,800
46 - 50	2,200	2,400	2,800
51 - 55	2,200	2,400	2,800
56 - 60	2,200	2,400	2,600
61 - 65	2,000	2,400	2,600
66 - 70	2,000	2,200	2,600
71 - 75	2,000	2,200	2,600
76+	2,000	2,200	2,400

SOURCE: USDA

Activity level	FEMALE		
	Sedentary	Moderately active	Active
Age (years)			
2	1,000	1,000	1,000
3	1,000	1,200	1,400
4	1,200	1,400	1,400
5	1,200	1,400	1,600
6	1,200	1,400	1,600
7	1,200	1,600	1,800
8	1,400	1,600	1,800
9	1,400	1,600	1,800
10	1,400	1,800	2,000
11	1,600	1,800	2,000
12	1,600	2,000	2,200
13	1,600	2,000	2,200
14	1,800	2,000	2,400
15	1,800	2,000	2,400
16	1,800	2,000	2,400
17	1,800	2,000	2,400
18	1,800	2,000	2,400
19 - 20	2,000	2,200	2,400
21 - 25	2,000	2,200	2,400
26 - 30	1,800	2,000	2,400
31 - 35	1,800	2,000	2,200
36 - 40	1,800	2,000	2,200
41 - 45	1,800	2,000	2,200
46 - 50	1,800	2,000	2,200
51 - 55	1,600	1,800	2,200
56 - 60	1,600	1,800	2,200
61 - 65	1,600	1,800	2,000
66 - 70	1,600	1,800	2,000
71 - 75	1,600	1,800	2,000
76+	1,600	1,800	2,000

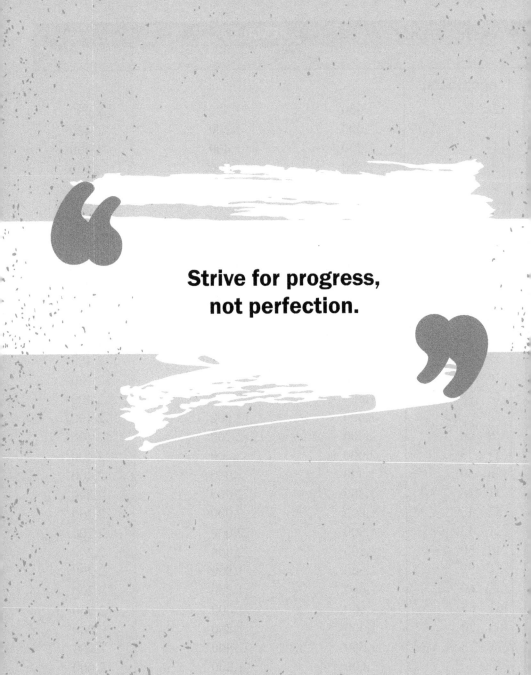

Strive for progress,
not perfection.

Body Mass Index

Body Mass Index (BMI)

BMI	19	20	21	22	23	24	25	26	27
Height (inches)	Body Weight (pounds)								
58	91	96	100	105	110	115	119	124	129
59	94	99	104	109	114	119	124	128	133
60	97	102	107	112	118	123	128	133	138
61	100	106	111	116	122	127	132	137	143
62	104	109	115	120	126	131	136	142	147
63	107	113	118	124	130	135	141	146	152
64	110	116	122	128	134	140	145	151	157
65	114	120	126	132	138	144	150	156	162
66	118	124	130	136	142	148	155	161	167
67	121	127	134	140	146	153	159	166	172
68	125	131	138	144	151	158	164	171	177
69	128	135	142	149	155	162	169	176	182
70	132	139	146	153	160	167	174	181	188
71	136	143	150	157	165	172	179	186	193
72	140	147	154	162	169	177	184	191	199
73	144	151	159	166	174	182	189	197	204
74	148	155	163	171	179	186	194	202	210
75	152	160	168	176	184	192	200	208	216
76	156	164	172	180	189	197	205	213	221

BMI RANGES

Underweight	Less than 18.5
Normal weight	18.5 - 24.9
Overweight	25 - 29.9
Obesity	30 or greater

SOURCE: U.S. DEPARTMENT OF HEALTH & HUMAN SERVICES

WEIGHT CONVERSION FORMULA

Pounds to Kilograms	lbs ÷ 2.2 = kilograms
Kilograms to Pounds	kg x 2.2 = pounds

28	29	30	31	32	33	34	35	36	37	38
Body Weight (pounds)										
134	138	143	148	153	158	162	167	172	177	181
138	143	148	153	158	163	168	173	178	183	188
143	148	153	158	163	168	174	179	184	189	194
148	153	158	164	169	174	180	185	190	195	201
153	158	164	169	175	180	186	191	196	202	207
158	163	169	175	180	186	191	197	203	208	214
163	169	174	180	186	192	197	204	209	215	221
168	174	180	186	192	198	204	210	216	222	228
173	179	186	192	198	204	210	216	223	229	235
178	185	191	198	204	211	217	223	230	236	242
184	190	197	203	210	216	223	230	236	243	249
189	196	203	209	216	223	230	236	243	250	257
195	202	209	216	222	229	236	243	250	257	264
200	208	215	222	229	236	243	250	257	265	272
206	213	221	228	235	242	250	258	265	272	279
212	219	227	235	242	250	257	265	272	280	288
218	225	233	241	249	256	264	272	280	287	295
224	232	240	248	256	264	272	279	287	295	303
230	238	246	254	263	271	279	287	295	304	312

Weight Conversion Table

kilograms (kg) to pounds (lb)

kg	lb	kg	lb	kg	lb	kg	lb
40	88	95	209	150	331	205	452
45	99	100	220	155	342	210	463
50	110	105	231	160	353	215	474
55	121	110	243	165	364	220	485
60	132	115	254	170	375	225	496
65	143	120	265	175	386	230	507
70	154	125	276	180	397	235	518
75	165	130	287	185	408	240	529
80	176	135	298	190	419	245	540
85	187	140	309	195	430	250	551
90	198	145	320	200	441	255	562

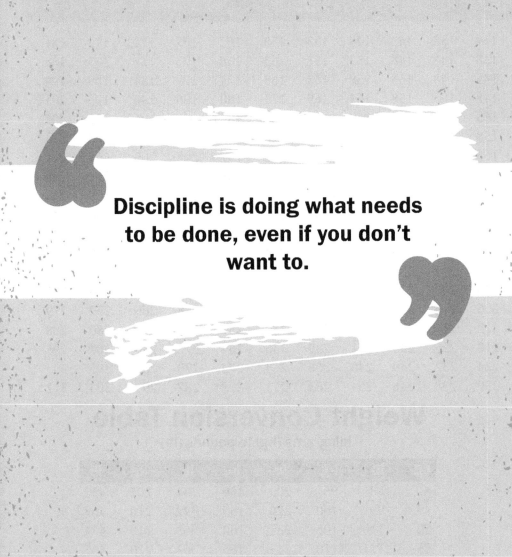

Discipline is doing what needs to be done, even if you don't want to.

Calorie Table of Common Foods

Calorie Table of Common Foods

(Nutrient amounts are listed in grams and rounded off)

FOOD	AMOUNT	CALS	FAT (SAT.)	CARBS	PROT.
DAIRY & EGGS					
Butter (salted)	1 tbsp	102	12 (7)	0	0
Cheese (cheddar)	1 tbsp	115	10 (5)	0	7
Cream (half and half)	1 cup	315	28 (17)	10	7
Sour Cream	1 cup	478	45 (40)	15	6
Milk (2%)	1 cup	122	5 (3)	12	8
Milk (1%)	1 cup	102	2 (2)	12	8
Yogourt (whole milk – plain)	1 cup	149	8 (5)	11	9
Yogourt (low fat – fruit)	1 cup	243	3 (2)	46	10
Egg (white)	1 large	17	0 (0)	0	4
Egg (whole – boiled)	1 large	78	5 (2)	1	6
Egg (whole – scrambled)	1 large	91	7 (2)	1	6
Egg (yolk)	1 large	55	5 (2)	1	3
Ice cream (soft serve – chocolate)	1 cup	382	22 (7)	38	7
Ice cream (fat-free)	1 cup	175	0 (0)	38	6
FATS & OILS					
Salad dressing (French)	1 tbsp	36	2 (0)	5	0
Salad dressing (Italian)	1 tbsp	35	3 (0)	2	0
Salad dressing (Ranch)	1 tbsp	63	7 (1)	1	0
Salad dressing (1000 Island)	1 tbsp	61	6 (1)	2	0
Oil (canola)	1 tbsp	124	14 (1)	0	0
Oil (coconut)	1 tbsp	117	14 (12)	0	0
Oil (olive)	1 tbsp	119	14 (2)	0	0
Oil (sunflower – high oleic, 70%+)	1 tbsp	124	14 (1)	0	0
Oil (vegetable)	1 tbsp	117	14 (11)	0	0
Margarine (with salt)	1 tbsp	100	11 (2)	0	0
Mayonnaise	1 tbsp	94	10 (2)	0	0
MEAT & FISH					
Beef (T-bone steak)	3 oz (85g)	190	13 (6)	0	17
Beef (rib eye)	3 oz (85g)	184	10 (4)	0	23
Beef (ribs)	3 oz (85g)	188	13 (5)	0	17
Chicken (fried - breaded)	3 oz (85g)	229	13 (4)	3	24
Chicken (breast – grilled)	3 oz (85g)	128	3 (1)	0	26

FOOD	AMOUNT	CALS	FAT (SAT.)	CARBS	PROT.
Corn (sweet)	1 med. (102g)	88	1 (0)	19	3
Fish (cod)	3 oz (85g)	89	1 (0)	0	19
Fish (halibut)	3 oz (85g)	94	1 (0)	0	19
Fish (salmon)	3 oz (85g)	121	5 (1)	0	17
Fish (tuna)	3 oz (85g)	73	1 (0)	0	17
Ham (lunch meat - sliced)	3 slices (3 oz)	138	15 (6)	6	15
Lamb (shoulder – whole)	3 oz (85g)	236	16 (7)	0	21
Pork (loin, whole)	3 oz (85g)	211	12 (5)	0	23
Roast beef (lunch meat - sliced)	3 slices (3 oz)	96	3 (0)	0	15
Salami (lunch meat - sliced)	3 slices (3 oz)	282	21 (9)	3	18
Sausage (Polish - smoked)	3 slices (3 oz)	252	21 (9)	3	9
Shrimp	3 oz (85g)	101	1 (0)	1	19
Turkey (lunch meat - sliced)	3 slices (3 oz.)	96	2 (1)	5	18
Turkey (roasted)	3 oz (85g)	102	10 (3)	0	15
Veal (shoulder, whole)	3 oz (85g)	111	4 (2)	0	16

MEALS

FOOD	AMOUNT	CALS	FAT (SAT.)	CARBS	PROT.
Chicken pot pie	1 pie (302g)	616	36 (13)	58	15
Chili (with beans)	1 cup (244g)	244	9 (3)	27	14
Egg rolls (chicken)	1 roll (80g)	158	4 (1)	23	8
Lasagna (with meat sauce)	1 piece (134g)	166	6 (3)	19	9
Macaroni and cheese	1 serving (244g)	200	6 (2)	28	8
Potato salad (with egg)	½ cup (125g)	196	12 (2)	20	2
Ravioli (cheese)	1 cup (242g)	186	4 (2)	33	6
Rice bowl (with chicken)	1 bowl (340g)	428	5 (1)	76	19
Spanish rice	1 cup (198g)	248	5 (1)	45	6
Turkey pot pie	397g	699	35 (11)	70	26
Spaghetti (with meatballs)	1 cup (246g)	246	10 (4)	28	11
Spaghettios (in meat sauce)	1 cup (252g)	174	2 (1)	31	8

CEREAL

FOOD	AMOUNT	CALS	FAT (SAT.)	CARBS	PROT.
All Bran	½ cup (31g)	81	2 (0)	23	4
Corn Flakes	1 cup (28g)	100	0 (0)	24	2
Cheerios	1 cup (28g)	105	2 (0)	21	3
Cream of wheat (salted)	1 cup	137	1 (0)	27	4
Kashi 7 Whole Grain Flakes	1 cup (50g)	168	1 (0)	41	6
Oats (quick)	1 cup	307	5 (1)	55	11
Quaker Instant Oatmeal (Cinnamon spice)	1 packet (43g)	159	2 (0)	32	4

FOOD	AMOUNT	CALS	FAT (SAT.	CARBS	PROT.
Raisin Bran	1 cup (59g)	191	1 (0)	47	4
Rice Krispies	1 cup (29g)	110	1 (0)	25	2
Shredded Wheat	1 cup (49g)	172	1 (0)	40	6

SOUP & SAUCES

FOOD	AMOUNT	CALS	FAT (SAT.	CARBS	PROT.
Campbell Red & White beef broth (condensed)	½ cup (124g)	15	0 (0)	1	3
Campbell Chunky chicken soup	1 cup (245g)	110	3 (1)	14	6
Chicken noodle soup	1 cup (245g)	56	1 (0)	9	2
Minestrone	1 cup (241g)	82	3 (1)	11	4
Cream of potato soup (with milk)	1 cup (248g)	149	6 (4)	17	6
Smart Soup (Thai Coconut Curry)	1 pouch (283g)	102	3 (1)	18	2
Tomato soup	1 cup (148g)	98	1 (0)	23	2
Vegetable beef soup	½ cup (126g)	79	2 (1)	10	6
Gravy (turkey)	1 cup	121	5 (1)	12	6

FRUIT & JUICES

FOOD	AMOUNT	CALS	FAT (SAT.	CARBS	PROT.
Apples	1 large	116	0 (0)	31	1
Apple juice	1 cup	114	0 (0)	28	0
Bananas	1 large	121	0 (0)	31	1
Blueberries	1 cup	84	0 (0)	21	1
Fig	1 fig	21	0 (0)	5	0
Fruit salad	1 cup	221	0 (0)	57	1
Orange (navel)	1 orange	69	0 (0)	18	1
Orange juice (concentrate)	1 cup	122	0 (0)	29	2
Peach	1 med.	58	0 (0)	14	1
Pear	1 med.	101	0 (0)	27	1
Raisins	1 cup	434	1 (0)	115	4
Strawberries	1 large	6	0 (0)	1	0

VEGETABLES

FOOD	AMOUNT	CALS	FAT (SAT.	CARBS	PROT.
Asparagus	1 cup	27	0 (0)	5	3
Beets	1 cup	58	0 (0)	13	2
Broccoli	1 cup	31	0 (0)	6	3
Carrots	1 medium	25	0 (0)	6	1
Celery	1 med. (40 g)		0 (0)	1	0

FOOD	AMOUNT	CALS	FAT (SAT.)	CARBS	PROT.
Cauliflower	1 cup (224g)	40	0 (0)	8	4
Celery	1 med. (40 g)	6	0 (0)	1	0
Cauliflower	1 cup (224g)	40	0 (0)	8	4
Corn (sweet)	1 med. (102g)	88	1 (0)	19	3
Eggplant	1 cup (82g)	20	0 (0)	5	1
Kale	1 cup (16g)	8	0 (0)	1	1
Leeks	1 cup (89g)	54	0 (0)	13	1
Lettuce	1 cup (36g)	5	0 (0)	1	0
Mushrooms (portabella – grilled)	1 cup (121g)	35	1 (0)	5	4
Mushrooms (white – raw)	1 cup (96g)	21	0 (0)	3	3
Onions (yellow – sauteed)	1 cup (87g)	115	9 (1)	7	1
Parsnips (cooked)	1 cup (156g)	111	0 (0)	27	2
Peas (green – cooked)	1 cup (160g)	134	0 (0)	25	9
Peppers (sweet – green)	1 cup (149g)	30	0 (0)	7	1
Potatoes (baked)	1 med. (173g)	168	0 (0)	37	5
Radishes	1 cup (116g)	19	0 (0)	4	1
Spinach	1 cup (30g)	7	0 (0)	1	1
Squash (butternut)	1 cup (205g)	82	0 (0)	22	2
Sweet potato	1 med. (114g)	103	0 (0)	24	2
Tomatoes	2 med. (246g)	44	0 (0)	10	2
Tomato juice	1 cup	41	1 (0)	9	2
Vegetables (mixed – frozen)	1 pkg (284g)	204	1 (0)	38	9
Yam	1 cup (136g)	158	0 (0)	37	2

BEANS/LEGUMES

FOOD	AMOUNT	CALS	FAT (SAT.)	CARBS	PROT.
Chickpeas	1 cup (164g)	269	4 (0)	45	15
Hummus	1 tbsp	27	1 (0)	3	1
Kidney beans	1 cup	53	1 (0)	8	8
Lentils	1 cup (77g)	82	0 (0)	17	7
Lima beans	1 cup	175	1 (0)	33	10
Peanuts (dry roasted, salted)	1 oz (28g)	166	14 (2)	6	7
Peanut butter	1 tbsp	191	16 (3)	7	7
Pinto beans	1 cup	275	1 (0)	53	16
Tofu	¼ block (81g)	57	3 (1)	1	7

GRAINS

FOOD	AMOUNT	CALS	FAT (SAT.)	CARBS	PROT.
Noodles (egg – cooked)	1 cup (160g)	221	3 (1)	40	7
Noodles (rice – cooked)	1 cup (176g)	190	0 (0)	42	3
Noodles (soba – cooked)	1 cup (114g)	113	0 (0)	24	6

FOOD	AMOUNT	CALS	FAT (SAT.)	CARBS	PROT.
Oats	1 cup (156g)	607	11 (2)	103	26
Rice (white – cooked)	1 cup (195g)	218	2 (0)	46	5
Spaghetti (wheat – cooked)	1 cup (140g)	221	1 (0)	438	

NUTS & SEEDS

FOOD	AMOUNT	CALS	FAT (SAT.)	CARBS	PROT.
Almonds	1 oz (28g)	164	14 (1)	6	6
Cashews	1 oz (28g)	157	12 (2)	9	5
Chia seeds	1 oz (28g)	138	9 (1)	12	5
Coconut (meat –raw)	1 med. (397g)	1405	132 (118)	60	13
Mixed nuts	1 oz (28g)	168	15 (2)	7	5
Pecans	1 oz (28g)	196	20 (2)	4	3
Pistachios	1 oz (28g)	159	13 (2)	8	6
Sunflower seeds (dry roasted – without salt)	1 oz (28g)	165	14 (1)	7	5
Walnuts	1 oz (28g)	185	18 (2)	4	4

BAKED GOODS

FOOD	AMOUNT	CALS	FAT (SAT.)	CARBS	PROT.
Bagel (plain)	1 med. (99g)	285	2 (0)	57	11
Bread (French or Vienna)	1 slice (139g)	378	3 (1)	72	15
Bread (pita – white)	1 large (60g)	165	1 (0)	33	5
Bread (dinner rolls)	1 piece (28g)	76	2 (0)	13	2
Bread (rye)	1 slice (24g)	68	1 (0)	13	2
Bread (whole wheat)	1 slice (32g)	81	1 (0)	14	4
Cake (sponge)	1 piece (63g)	187	3 (1)	36	5
Cookies (chocolate chip)	¼ pkg (124g)	616	31 (10)	82	6
Cookies (oatmeal)	¼ pkg (124g)	573	24 (6)	83	8
Crackers (wheat)	16 pcs (34g)	155	6 (1)	24	2
Croissants (butter)	1 med. (57g)	231	12 (7)	26	5
Doughnuts (plain)	1 med. (45g)	192	10 (3)	23	2
Eggo waffles	2 waffles (70g)	141	2 (1)	27	5
English muffins	1 piece (57g)	127	1 (0)	25	5
French toast	1 slice (65g)	149	7 (2)	16	5
Pancakes	1 piece (41g)	96	3 (1)	15	2
Pie (apple)	1 piece (155g)	411	19 (5)	58	4
Waffles	1 piece (39g)	106	4 (1)	16	3

FAST FOOD

FOOD	AMOUNT	CALS	FAT (SAT.)	CARBS	PROT.
Burritos (with beef)	2 pieces	524	21 (10)	59	27
Cheeseburger (single – plain)	1 burger (91g)	280	13 (6)	26	15
Hamburger (single – plain)	1 burger (78g)	232	9 (4)	25	13

FOOD	AMOUNT	CALS	FAT (SAT.	CARBS	PROT.
Hotdog (plain)	1 hotdog (98g)	242	15 (5)	18	10
Nachos (with cheese)	1 serving (80g)	274	17 (2)	28	3
Pizza (cheese)	1 slice (76g)	230	10 (5)	24	10
Fried chicken (wing – breaded)	1 wing (58g)	180	12 (3)	7	12

SNACKS & SWEETS

FOOD	AMOUNT	CALS	FAT (SAT.	CARBS	PROT.
Chewing gum	1 stick (3g)	11	0 (0)	3	0
Chocolate	¼ bar (28g)	162	11 (6)	15	2
Frozen yogourt	½ cup (72g)	115	4 (3)	18	3
Fruit & juice bars	1 bar (77g)	67	0 (0)	16	1
Fudgsicle	1 serving (84g)	88	1 (0)	19	3
Granola bars	1 bar (25g)	118	5 (1)	16	3
Kit Kat	1 bar (42g)	218	11 (8)	27	3
Reese Peanut Butter Cups	1 bar (45g)	232	14 (5)	25	5
Skittles (Original)	1 pack (62g)	251	3 (3)	56	0
Snickers	1 bar (57g)	280	14 (5)	35	4
Popcorn	1 cup (8g)	31	0 (0)	6	1
Pop Tarts	1 pastry (52g)	207	5 (2)	37	2
Potato chips (plain – salted)	¼ bag (57g)	304	20 (3)	30	4
Rice cakes	2 cakes (18g)	71	1 (0)	15	1
Tortilla chips	¼ bag (53g)	251	11 (1)	36	4
Trail mix	½ cup (75g)	346	22 (4)	34	10
Pudding (chocolate)	1 serving (25g)	94	0 (0)	22	1
Sundae (hot fudge)	1 sundae (158g)	284	9 (5)	48	6

BEVERAGES

FOOD	AMOUNT	CALS	FAT (SAT.	CARBS	PROT.
Beer	1 can (12 oz)	153	0	13	2
Coconut water	1 cup	46	0 (0)	9	2
Coffee (brewed – grounds)	1 cup	2	0	0	0
Cola	1 can (12 oz)	152	0	39	0
Soy milk (Silk)	1 cup (243g)	100	4 (1)	8	7
Tea (black)	1 cup	2	0	1	0
Vodka	1 shot (1.5 oz)	97	0	0	0
Water	1 cup	0	0	0	0
Wine (red)	1 glass (5 oz)	125	0	4	0
Wine (white)	1 glass (5 oz)	118	0	6	0

SOURCE: USDA

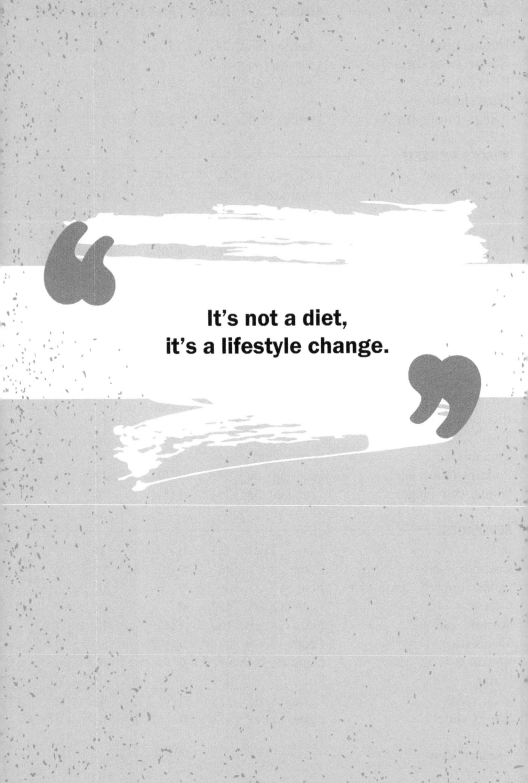

It's not a diet,
it's a lifestyle change.

Weight Loss Log

Weight Loss Log

Start Date: _____ Start Weight: _____ Goal Weight: _____

Starting Measurements

Chest: _____ Waist: _____ Thigh: _____ Arm: _____

| DATE | WEIGHT | WEEKLY WEIGHT LOSS | CUMULA-TIVE WEIGHT LOSS | MEASUREMENTS | | | | WEEKLY INCH LOSS | CUMU-LATIVE INCH LOSS |
				CHEST	WAIST	THIGH	ARM		

DATE	WEIGHT	WEEKLY WEIGHT LOSS	CUMULA-TIVE WEIGHT LOSS	MEASUREMENTS				WEEKLY INCH LOSS	CUMU-LATIVE INCH LOSS
				CHEST	WAIST	THIGH	ARM		

DATE	WEIGHT	WEEKLY WEIGHT LOSS	CUMULA-TIVE WEIGHT LOSS	MEASUREMENTS				WEEKLY INCH LOSS	CUMU-LATIVE INCH LOSS
				CHEST	WAIST	THIGH	ARM		

| DATE | WEIGHT | WEEKLY WEIGHT LOSS | CUMULA-TIVE WEIGHT LOSS | MEASUREMENTS | | | | WEEKLY INCH LOSS | CUMU-LATIVE INCH LOSS |
				CHEST	WAIST	THIGH	ARM		

Be stronger than your excuses.

Food Journal

Food Journal

DATE			WATER (# glasses)		WEIGHT	
	Calories	Fat	Carbs	Protein	Notes	
B'fast						
Lunch						
Dinner						
Snack						
TOTALS						

DATE			WATER (# glasses)		WEIGHT	
	Calories	Fat	Carbs	Protein	Notes	
B'fast						
Lunch						
Dinner						
Snack						
TOTALS						

DATE			WATER (# glasses)		WEIGHT	
	Calories	Fat	Carbs	Protein	Notes	
B'fast						
Lunch						
Dinner						
Snack						
TOTALS						

DATE			WATER (# glasses)		WEIGHT	
	Calories	Fat	Carbs	Protein		Notes
B'fast						
Lunch						
Dinner						
Snack						
TOTALS						

DATE			WATER (# glasses)		WEIGHT	
	Calories	Fat	Carbs	Protein		Notes
B'fast						
Lunch						
Dinner						
Snack						
TOTALS						

DATE			WATER (# glasses)		WEIGHT	
	Calories	Fat	Carbs	Protein		Notes
B'fast						
Lunch						
Dinner						
Snack						
TOTALS						

DATE			WATER (# glasses)		WEIGHT	
	Calories	Fat	Carbs	Protein	Notes	
B'fast						
Lunch						
Dinner						
Snack						
TOTALS						

DATE			WATER (# glasses)		WEIGHT	
	Calories	Fat	Carbs	Protein	Notes	
B'fast						
Lunch						
Dinner						
Snack						
TOTALS						

DATE			WATER (# glasses)		WEIGHT	
	Calories	Fat	Carbs	Protein	Notes	
B'fast						
Lunch						
Dinner						
Snack						
TOTALS						

DATE			WATER (# glasses)		WEIGHT	
	Calories	Fat	Carbs	Protein	Notes	
B'fast						
Lunch						
Dinner						
Snack						
TOTALS						

DATE			WATER (# glasses)		WEIGHT	
	Calories	Fat	Carbs	Protein	Notes	
B'fast						
Lunch						
Dinner						
Snack						
TOTALS						

DATE			WATER (# glasses)		WEIGHT	
	Calories	Fat	Carbs	Protein	Notes	
B'fast						
Lunch						
Dinner						
Snack						
TOTALS						

DATE			WATER (# glasses)		WEIGHT	
	Calories	Fat	Carbs	Protein	Notes	
B'fast						
Lunch						
Dinner						
Snack						
TOTALS						

DATE			WATER (# glasses)		WEIGHT	
	Calories	Fat	Carbs	Protein	Notes	
B'fast						
Lunch						
Dinner						
Snack						
TOTALS						

DATE			WATER (# glasses)		WEIGHT	
	Calories	Fat	Carbs	Protein	Notes	
B'fast						
Lunch						
Dinner						
Snack						
TOTALS						

DATE			WATER (# glasses)		WEIGHT	
	Calories	Fat	Carbs	Protein	Notes	
B'fast						
Lunch						
Dinner						
Snack						
TOTALS						

DATE			WATER (# glasses)		WEIGHT	
	Calories	Fat	Carbs	Protein	Notes	
B'fast						
Lunch						
Dinner						
Snack						
TOTALS						

DATE			WATER (# glasses)		WEIGHT	
	Calories	Fat	Carbs	Protein	Notes	
B'fast						
Lunch						
Dinner						
Snack						
TOTALS						

DATE			WATER (# glasses)		WEIGHT	
	Calories	Fat	Carbs	Protein	Notes	
B'fast						
Lunch						
Dinner						
Snack						
TOTALS						

DATE			WATER (# glasses)		WEIGHT	
	Calories	Fat	Carbs	Protein	Notes	
B'fast						
Lunch						
Dinner						
Snack						
TOTALS						

DATE			WATER (# glasses)		WEIGHT	
	Calories	Fat	Carbs	Protein	Notes	
B'fast						
Lunch						
Dinner						
Snack						
TOTALS						

DATE			WATER (# glasses)		WEIGHT	
	Calories	Fat	Carbs	Protein	Notes	
B'fast						
Lunch						
Dinner						
Snack						
TOTALS						

DATE			WATER (# glasses)		WEIGHT	
	Calories	Fat	Carbs	Protein	Notes	
B'fast						
Lunch						
Dinner						
Snack						
TOTALS						

DATE			WATER (# glasses)		WEIGHT	
	Calories	Fat	Carbs	Protein	Notes	
B'fast						
Lunch						
Dinner						
Snack						
TOTALS						

DATE			WATER (# glasses)		WEIGHT	
	Calories	Fat	Carbs	Protein	Notes	
B'fast						
Lunch						
Dinner						
Snack						
TOTALS						

DATE			WATER (# glasses)		WEIGHT	
	Calories	Fat	Carbs	Protein	Notes	
B'fast						
Lunch						
Dinner						
Snack						
TOTALS						

DATE			WATER (# glasses)		WEIGHT	
	Calories	Fat	Carbs	Protein	Notes	
B'fast						
Lunch						
Dinner						
Snack						
TOTALS						

DATE			WATER (# glasses)		WEIGHT	
	Calories	Fat	Carbs	Protein	Notes	
B'fast						
Lunch						
Dinner						
Snack						
TOTALS						

DATE			WATER (# glasses)		WEIGHT	
	Calories	Fat	Carbs	Protein	Notes	
B'fast						
Lunch						
Dinner						
Snack						
TOTALS						

DATE			WATER (# glasses)		WEIGHT	
	Calories	Fat	Carbs	Protein	Notes	
B'fast						
Lunch						
Dinner						
Snack						
TOTALS						

DATE			WATER (# glasses)		WEIGHT	
	Calories	Fat	Carbs	Protein	Notes	
B'fast						
Lunch						
Dinner						
Snack						
TOTALS						

DATE			WATER (# glasses)		WEIGHT	
	Calories	Fat	Carbs	Protein	Notes	
B'fast						
Lunch						
Dinner						
Snack						
TOTALS						

DATE			WATER (# glasses)		WEIGHT	
	Calories	Fat	Carbs	Protein	Notes	
B'fast						
Lunch						
Dinner						
Snack						
TOTALS						

DATE			WATER (# glasses)		WEIGHT	
	Calories	Fat	Carbs	Protein	Notes	
B'fast						
Lunch						
Dinner						
Snack						
TOTALS						

DATE			WATER (# glasses)		WEIGHT	
	Calories	Fat	Carbs	Protein	Notes	
B'fast						
Lunch						
Dinner						
Snack						
TOTALS						

DATE			WATER (# glasses)		WEIGHT	
	Calories	Fat	Carbs	Protein	Notes	
B'fast						
Lunch						
Dinner						
Snack						
TOTALS						

DATE			WATER (# glasses)		WEIGHT	
	Calories	Fat	Carbs	Protein	Notes	
B'fast						
Lunch						
Dinner						
Snack						
TOTALS						

DATE			WATER (# glasses)		WEIGHT	
	Calories	Fat	Carbs	Protein	Notes	
B'fast						
Lunch						
Dinner						
Snack						
TOTALS						

DATE			WATER (# glasses)		WEIGHT	
	Calories	Fat	Carbs	Protein	Notes	
B'fast						
Lunch						
Dinner						
Snack						
TOTALS						

DATE			WATER (# glasses)		WEIGHT	
	Calories	Fat	Carbs	Protein	Notes	
B'fast						
Lunch						
Dinner						
Snack						
TOTALS						

DATE			WATER (# glasses)		WEIGHT	
	Calories	Fat	Carbs	Protein	Notes	
B'fast						
Lunch						
Dinner						
Snack						
TOTALS						

DATE			WATER (# glasses)		WEIGHT	
	Calories	Fat	Carbs	Protein	Notes	
B'fast						
Lunch						
Dinner						
Snack						
TOTALS						

DATE			WATER (# glasses)		WEIGHT	
	Calories	Fat	Carbs	Protein	Notes	
B'fast						
Lunch						
Dinner						
Snack						
TOTALS						

DATE			WATER (# glasses)		WEIGHT	
	Calories	Fat	Carbs	Protein	Notes	
B'fast						
Lunch						
Dinner						
Snack						
TOTALS						

DATE			WATER (# glasses)		WEIGHT	
	Calories	Fat	Carbs	Protein	Notes	
B'fast						
Lunch						
Dinner						
Snack						
TOTALS						

DATE			WATER (# glasses)		WEIGHT	
	Calories	Fat	Carbs	Protein	Notes	
B'fast						
Lunch						
Dinner						
Snack						
TOTALS						

DATE			WATER (# glasses)		WEIGHT	
	Calories	Fat	Carbs	Protein	Notes	
B'fast						
Lunch						
Dinner						
Snack						
TOTALS						

DATE			WATER (# glasses)		WEIGHT	
	Calories	Fat	Carbs	Protein	Notes	
B'fast						
Lunch						
Dinner						
Snack						
TOTALS						

DATE			WATER (# glasses)		WEIGHT	
	Calories	Fat	Carbs	Protein	Notes	
B'fast						
Lunch						
Dinner						
Snack						
TOTALS						

DATE			WATER (# glasses)		WEIGHT	
	Calories	Fat	Carbs	Protein	Notes	
B'fast						
Lunch						
Dinner						
Snack						
TOTALS						

DATE			WATER (# glasses)		WEIGHT	
	Calories	Fat	Carbs	Protein	Notes	
B'fast						
Lunch						
Dinner						
Snack						
TOTALS						

DATE			WATER (# glasses)		WEIGHT	
	Calories	Fat	Carbs	Protein	Notes	
B'fast						
Lunch						
Dinner						
Snack						
TOTALS						

DATE			WATER (# glasses)		WEIGHT	
	Calories	Fat	Carbs	Protein	Notes	
B'fast						
Lunch						
Dinner						
Snack						
TOTALS						

DATE			WATER (# glasses)		WEIGHT	
	Calories	Fat	Carbs	Protein	Notes	
B'fast						
Lunch						
Dinner						
Snack						
TOTALS						

DATE			WATER (# glasses)		WEIGHT	
	Calories	Fat	Carbs	Protein	Notes	
B'fast						
Lunch						
Dinner						
Snack						
TOTALS						

DATE			WATER (# glasses)		WEIGHT	
	Calories	Fat	Carbs	Protein	Notes	
B'fast						
Lunch						
Dinner						
Snack						
TOTALS						

DATE			WATER (# glasses)		WEIGHT	
	Calories	Fat	Carbs	Protein	Notes	
B'fast						
Lunch						
Dinner						
Snack						
TOTALS						

DATE			WATER (# glasses)		WEIGHT	
	Calories	Fat	Carbs	Protein	Notes	
B'fast						
Lunch						
Dinner						
Snack						
TOTALS						

DATE			WATER (# glasses)		WEIGHT	
	Calories	Fat	Carbs	Protein	Notes	
B'fast						
Lunch						
Dinner						
Snack						
TOTALS						

DATE			WATER (# glasses)		WEIGHT	
	Calories	Fat	Carbs	Protein	Notes	
B'fast						
Lunch						
Dinner						
Snack						
TOTALS						

DATE			WATER (# glasses)		WEIGHT	
	Calories	Fat	Carbs	Protein	Notes	
B'fast						
Lunch						
Dinner						
Snack						
TOTALS						

DATE			WATER (# glasses)		WEIGHT	
	Calories	Fat	Carbs	Protein	Notes	
B'fast						
Lunch						
Dinner						
Snack						
TOTALS						

DATE			WATER (# glasses)		WEIGHT	
	Calories	Fat	Carbs	Protein	Notes	
B'fast						
Lunch						
Dinner						
Snack						
TOTALS						

DATE			WATER (# glasses)		WEIGHT	
	Calories	Fat	Carbs	Protein	Notes	
B'fast						
Lunch						
Dinner						
Snack						
TOTALS						

DATE			WATER (# glasses)		WEIGHT	
	Calories	Fat	Carbs	Protein	Notes	
B'fast						
Lunch						
Dinner						
Snack						
TOTALS						

DATE			WATER (# glasses)		WEIGHT	
	Calories	Fat	Carbs	Protein	Notes	
B'fast						
Lunch						
Dinner						
Snack						
TOTALS						

DATE			WATER (# glasses)		WEIGHT	
	Calories	Fat	Carbs	Protein	Notes	
B'fast						
Lunch						
Dinner						
Snack						
TOTALS						

DATE			WATER (# glasses)		WEIGHT	
	Calories	Fat	Carbs	Protein	Notes	
B'fast						
Lunch						
Dinner						
Snack						
TOTALS						

DATE			WATER (# glasses)		WEIGHT	
	Calories	Fat	Carbs	Protein	Notes	
B'fast						
Lunch						
Dinner						
Snack						
TOTALS						

DATE			WATER (# glasses)		WEIGHT	
	Calories	Fat	Carbs	Protein	Notes	
B'fast						
Lunch						
Dinner						
Snack						
TOTALS						

DATE			WATER (# glasses)		WEIGHT	
	Calories	Fat	Carbs	Protein	Notes	
B'fast						
Lunch						
Dinner						
Snack						
TOTALS						

DATE			WATER (# glasses)		WEIGHT	
	Calories	Fat	Carbs	Protein	Notes	
B'fast						
Lunch						
Dinner						
Snack						
TOTALS						

DATE			WATER (# glasses)		WEIGHT	
	Calories	Fat	Carbs	Protein	Notes	
B'fast						
Lunch						
Dinner						
Snack						
TOTALS						

DATE			WATER (# glasses)		WEIGHT	
	Calories	Fat	Carbs	Protein	Notes	
B'fast						
Lunch						
Dinner						
Snack						
TOTALS						

DATE			WATER (# glasses)		WEIGHT	
	Calories	Fat	Carbs	Protein	Notes	
B'fast						
Lunch						
Dinner						
Snack						
TOTALS						

DATE			WATER (# glasses)		WEIGHT	
	Calories	Fat	Carbs	Protein	Notes	
B'fast						
Lunch						
Dinner						
Snack						
TOTALS						

DATE			WATER (# glasses)		WEIGHT	
	Calories	Fat	Carbs	Protein	Notes	
B'fast						
Lunch						
Dinner						
Snack						
TOTALS						

DATE			WATER (# glasses)		WEIGHT	
	Calories	Fat	Carbs	Protein	Notes	
B'fast						
Lunch						
Dinner						
Snack						
TOTALS						

DATE			WATER (# glasses)		WEIGHT	
	Calories	Fat	Carbs	Protein	Notes	
B'fast						
Lunch						
Dinner						
Snack						
TOTALS						

DATE			WATER (# glasses)		WEIGHT	
	Calories	Fat	Carbs	Protein	Notes	
B'fast						
Lunch						
Dinner						
Snack						
TOTALS						

DATE			WATER (# glasses)		WEIGHT	
	Calories	Fat	Carbs	Protein	Notes	
B'fast						
Lunch						
Dinner						
Snack						
TOTALS						

DATE			WATER (# glasses)		WEIGHT	
	Calories	Fat	Carbs	Protein	Notes	
B'fast						
Lunch						
Dinner						
Snack						
TOTALS						

DATE			WATER (# glasses)		WEIGHT	
	Calories	Fat	Carbs	Protein	Notes	
B'fast						
Lunch						
Dinner						
Snack						
TOTALS						

DATE			WATER (# glasses)		WEIGHT	
	Calories	Fat	Carbs	Protein	Notes	
B'fast						
Lunch						
Dinner						
Snack						
TOTALS						

DATE			WATER (# glasses)		WEIGHT	
	Calories	Fat	Carbs	Protein	Notes	
B'fast						
Lunch						
Dinner						
Snack						
TOTALS						

DATE			WATER (# glasses)		WEIGHT	
	Calories	Fat	Carbs	Protein	Notes	
B'fast						
Lunch						
Dinner						
Snack						
TOTALS						

DATE			WATER (# glasses)		WEIGHT	
	Calories	Fat	Carbs	Protein	Notes	
B'fast						
Lunch						
Dinner						
Snack						
TOTALS						

DATE			WATER (# glasses)		WEIGHT	
	Calories	Fat	Carbs	Protein	Notes	
B'fast						
Lunch						
Dinner						
Snack						
TOTALS						

DATE			WATER (# glasses)		WEIGHT	
	Calories	Fat	Carbs	Protein	Notes	
B'fast						
Lunch						
Dinner						
Snack						
TOTALS						

DATE			WATER (# glasses)		WEIGHT	
	Calories	Fat	Carbs	Protein	Notes	
B'fast						
Lunch						
Dinner						
Snack						
TOTALS						

DATE			WATER (# glasses)		WEIGHT	
	Calories	Fat	Carbs	Protein	Notes	
B'fast						
Lunch						
Dinner						
Snack						
TOTALS						

DATE			WATER (# glasses)		WEIGHT	
	Calories	Fat	Carbs	Protein	Notes	
B'fast						
Lunch						
Dinner						
Snack						
TOTALS						

DATE			WATER (# glasses)		WEIGHT	
	Calories	Fat	Carbs	Protein	Notes	
B'fast						
Lunch						
Dinner						
Snack						
TOTALS						

DATE			WATER (# glasses)		WEIGHT	
	Calories	Fat	Carbs	Protein	Notes	
B'fast						
Lunch						
Dinner						
Snack						
TOTALS						

DATE			WATER (# glasses)		WEIGHT	
	Calories	Fat	Carbs	Protein	Notes	
B'fast						
Lunch						
Dinner						
Snack						
TOTALS						

DATE			WATER (# glasses)		WEIGHT	
	Calories	Fat	Carbs	Protein	Notes	
B'fast						
Lunch						
Dinner						
Snack						
TOTALS						

DATE			WATER (# glasses)		WEIGHT	
	Calories	Fat	Carbs	Protein	Notes	
B'fast						
Lunch						
Dinner						
Snack						
TOTALS						

DATE			WATER (# glasses)		WEIGHT	
	Calories	Fat	Carbs	Protein	Notes	
B'fast						
Lunch						
Dinner						
Snack						
TOTALS						

DATE			WATER (# glasses)		WEIGHT	
	Calories	Fat	Carbs	Protein	Notes	
B'fast						
Lunch						
Dinner						
Snack						
TOTALS						

DATE			WATER (# glasses)		WEIGHT	
	Calories	Fat	Carbs	Protein	Notes	
B'fast						
Lunch						
Dinner						
Snack						
TOTALS						

DATE			WATER (# glasses)		WEIGHT	
	Calories	Fat	Carbs	Protein	Notes	
B'fast						
Lunch						
Dinner						
Snack						
TOTALS						

DATE			WATER (# glasses)		WEIGHT	
	Calories	Fat	Carbs	Protein	Notes	
B'fast						
Lunch						
Dinner						
Snack						
TOTALS						

DATE			WATER (# glasses)		WEIGHT	
	Calories	Fat	Carbs	Protein	Notes	
B'fast						
Lunch						
Dinner						
Snack						
TOTALS						

DATE			WATER (# glasses)		WEIGHT	
	Calories	Fat	Carbs	Protein	Notes	
B'fast						
Lunch						
Dinner						
Snack						
TOTALS						

DATE			WATER (# glasses)		WEIGHT	
	Calories	Fat	Carbs	Protein	Notes	
B'fast						
Lunch						
Dinner						
Snack						
TOTALS						

DATE			WATER (# glasses)		WEIGHT	
	Calories	Fat	Carbs	Protein	Notes	
B'fast						
Lunch						
Dinner						
Snack						
TOTALS						

DATE			WATER (# glasses)		WEIGHT	
	Calories	Fat	Carbs	Protein	Notes	
B'fast						
Lunch						
Dinner						
Snack						
TOTALS						

DATE			WATER (# glasses)		WEIGHT	
	Calories	Fat	Carbs	Protein	Notes	
B'fast						
Lunch						
Dinner						
Snack						
TOTALS						

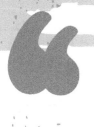

Life is 10% what happens to me and 90% of how I react to it.

CHARLES SWINDOLL

Medication and Supplement Lists

Medications List

Medication	Dose	Frequency	Time taken	Taken for	Date started	Prescribed by

Nutritional Supplements List

Medication	Dose	Frequency	Time taken	Taken for	Date started	Prescribed by

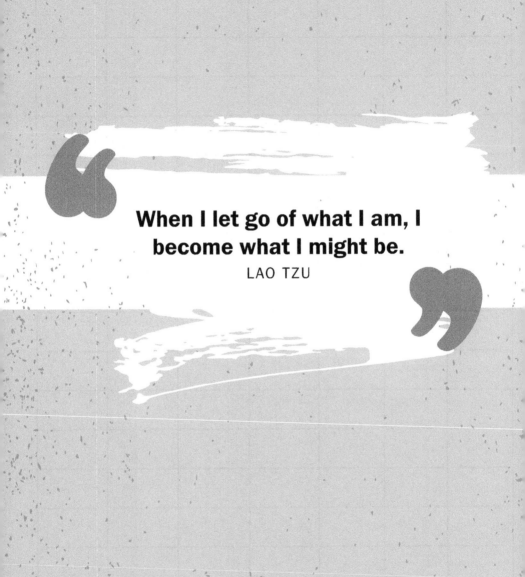

When I let go of what I am, I become what I might be.

LAO TZU

Blood Glucose Log

Blood Glucose Log

DATE	BREAKFAST		MEDICINE	LUNCH		MEDICINE	DINNER		MEDICINE
	Before	2h after		Before	2h after		Before	2h after	

SNACK		MEDICINE	BEDTIME	NIGHT	EXERCISE	STRESS	SLEEP	NOTES
Before	2h after							

DATE	BREAKFAST		MEDICINE	LUNCH		MEDICINE	DINNER		MEDICINE
	Before	2h after		Before	2h after		Before	2h after	

SNACK			MEDICINE	BEDTIME	NIGHT	EXERCISE	STRESS	SLEEP		NOTES
Before	2h after									

DATE	BREAKFAST		MEDICINE	LUNCH		MEDICINE	DINNER		MEDICINE
	Before	2h after		Before	2h after		Before	2h after	

SNACK		MEDICINE	BEDTIME	NIGHT	EXERCISE	STRESS	SLEEP	NOTES
Before	2h after							

DATE	BREAKFAST		MEDICINE	LUNCH		MEDICINE	DINNER		MEDICINE
	Before	2h after		Before	2h after		Before	2h after	

SNACK		MEDICINE	BEDTIME	NIGHT	EXERCISE	STRESS	SLEEP	NOTES
Before	2h after							

DATE	BREAKFAST		MEDICINE	LUNCH		MEDICINE	DINNER		MEDICINE
	Before	2h after		Before	2h after		Before	2h after	

SNACK		MEDICINE	BEDTIME	NIGHT	EXERCISE	STRESS	SLEEP	NOTES
Before	2h after							

DATE	BREAKFAST		MEDICINE	LUNCH		MEDICINE	DINNER		MEDICINE
	Before	2h after		Before	2h after		Before	2h after	

SNACK		MEDICINE	BEDTIME	NIGHT	EXERCISE	STRESS	SLEEP	NOTES
Before	2h after							

DATE	BREAKFAST		MEDICINE	LUNCH		MEDICINE	DINNER		MEDICINE
	Before	2h after		Before	2h after		Before	2h after	

SNACK		MEDICINE	BEDTIME	NIGHT	EXERCISE	STRESS	SLEEP	NOTES
Before	2h after							

DATE	BREAKFAST		MEDICINE	LUNCH		MEDICINE	DINNER		MEDICINE
	Before	2h after		Before	2h after		Before	2h after	

SNACK		MEDICINE	BEDTIME	NIGHT	EXERCISE	STRESS	SLEEP	NOTES
Before	2h after							

DATE	BREAKFAST		MEDICINE	LUNCH		MEDICINE	DINNER		MEDICINE
	Before	2h after		Before	2h after		Before	2h after	

SNACK		MEDICINE	BEDTIME	NIGHT	EXERCISE	STRESS	SLEEP	NOTES
Before	2h after							

DATE	BREAKFAST		MEDICINE	LUNCH		MEDICINE	DINNER		MEDICINE
	Before	2h after		Before	2h after		Before	2h after	

SNACK		MEDICINE	BEDTIME	NIGHT	EXERCISE	STRESS	SLEEP	NOTES
Before	2h after							

DATE	BREAKFAST		MEDICINE	LUNCH		MEDICINE	DINNER		MEDICINE
	Before	2h after		Before	2h after		Before	2h after	

SNACK		MEDICINE	BEDTIME	NIGHT	EXERCISE	STRESS	SLEEP	NOTES
Before	2h after							

DATE	BREAKFAST		MEDICINE	LUNCH		MEDICINE	DINNER		MEDICINE
	Before	2h after		Before	2h after		Before	2h after	

SNACK		MEDICINE	BEDTIME	NIGHT	EXERCISE	STRESS	SLEEP	NOTES
Before	2h after							

DATE	BREAKFAST		MEDICINE	LUNCH		MEDICINE	DINNER		MEDICINE
	Before	2h after		Before	2h after		Before	2h after	

SNACK		MEDICINE	BEDTIME	NIGHT	EXERCISE	STRESS	SLEEP	NOTES
Before	2h after							

DATE	BREAKFAST		MEDICINE	LUNCH		MEDICINE	DINNER		MEDICINE
	Before	2h after		Before	2h after		Before	2h after	

SNACK		MEDICINE	BEDTIME	NIGHT	EXERCISE	STRESS	SLEEP	NOTES
Before	2h after							

DATE	BREAKFAST		MEDICINE	LUNCH		MEDICINE	DINNER		MEDICINE
	Before	2h after		Before	2h after		Before	2h after	

SNACK		MEDICINE	BEDTIME	NIGHT	EXERCISE	STRESS	SLEEP	NOTES
Before	2h after							

DATE	BREAKFAST		MEDICINE	LUNCH		MEDICINE	DINNER		MEDICINE
	Before	2h after		Before	2h after		Before	2h after	

SNACK		MEDICINE	BEDTIME	NIGHT	EXERCISE	STRESS	SLEEP	NOTES
Before	2h after							

DATE	BREAKFAST		MEDICINE	LUNCH		MEDICINE	DINNER		MEDICINE
	Before	2h after		Before	2h after		Before	2h after	

SNACK		MEDICINE	BEDTIME	NIGHT	EXERCISE	STRESS	SLEEP	NOTES
Before	2h after							

DATE	BREAKFAST		MEDICINE	LUNCH		MEDICINE	DINNER		MEDICINE
	Before	2h after		Before	2h after		Before	2h after	

SNACK		MEDICINE	BEDTIME	NIGHT	EXERCISE	STRESS	SLEEP	NOTES
Before	2h after							

DATE	BREAKFAST		MEDICINE	LUNCH		MEDICINE	DINNER		MEDICINE
	Before	2h after		Before	2h after		Before	2h after	

	SNACK		MEDICINE	BEDTIME	NIGHT	EXERCISE	STRESS	SLEEP	NOTES
	Before	2h after							

DATE	BREAKFAST		MEDICINE	LUNCH		MEDICINE	DINNER		MEDICINE
	Before	2h after		Before	2h after		Before	2h after	

SNACK		MEDICINE	BEDTIME	NIGHT	EXERCISE	STRESS	SLEEP	NOTES
Before	2h after							

DATE	BREAKFAST		MEDICINE	LUNCH		MEDICINE	DINNER		MEDICINE
	Before	2h after		Before	2h after		Before	2h after	

SNACK		MEDICINE	BEDTIME	NIGHT	EXERCISE	STRESS	SLEEP	NOTES
Before	2h after							

DATE	BREAKFAST		MEDICINE	LUNCH		MEDICINE	DINNER		MEDICINE
	Before	2h after		Before	2h after		Before	2h after	

	SNACK		MEDICINE	BEDTIME	NIGHT	EXERCISE	STRESS	SLEEP	NOTES
	Before	2h after							

DATE	BREAKFAST		MEDICINE	LUNCH		MEDICINE	DINNER		MEDICINE
	Before	2h after		Before	2h after		Before	2h after	

SNACK		MEDICINE	BEDTIME	NIGHT	EXERCISE	STRESS	SLEEP	NOTES
Before	2h after							

DATE	BREAKFAST		MEDICINE	LUNCH		MEDICINE	DINNER		MEDICINE
	Before	2h after		Before	2h after		Before	2h after	

SNACK		MEDICINE	BEDTIME	NIGHT	EXERCISE	STRESS	SLEEP	NOTES
Before	2h after							

DATE	BREAKFAST		MEDICINE	LUNCH		MEDICINE	DINNER		MEDICINE
	Before	2h after		Before	2h after		Before	2h after	

SNACK		MEDICINE	BEDTIME	NIGHT	EXERCISE	STRESS	SLEEP	NOTES
Before	2h after							

DATE	BREAKFAST		MEDICINE	LUNCH		MEDICINE	DINNER		MEDICINE
	Before	2h after		Before	2h after		Before	2h after	

SNACK		MEDICINE	BEDTIME	NIGHT	EXERCISE	STRESS	SLEEP	NOTES
Before	2h after							

DATE	BREAKFAST		MEDICINE	LUNCH		MEDICINE	DINNER		MEDICINE
	Before	2h after		Before	2h after		Before	2h after	

SNACK		MEDICINE	BEDTIME	NIGHT	EXERCISE	STRESS	SLEEP	NOTES
Before	2h after							

DATE	BREAKFAST		MEDICINE	LUNCH		MEDICINE	DINNER		MEDICINE
	Before	2h after		Before	2h after		Before	2h after	

SNACK		MEDICINE	BEDTIME	NIGHT	EXERCISE	STRESS	SLEEP	NOTES
Before	2h after							

DATE	BREAKFAST		MEDICINE	LUNCH		MEDICINE	DINNER		MEDICINE
	Before	2h after		Before	2h after		Before	2h after	

SNACK		MEDICINE	BEDTIME	NIGHT	EXERCISE	STRESS	SLEEP	NOTES
Before	2h after							

DATE	BREAKFAST		MEDICINE	LUNCH		MEDICINE	DINNER		MEDICINE
	Before	2h after		Before	2h after		Before	2h after	

SNACK		MEDICINE	BEDTIME	NIGHT	EXERCISE	STRESS	SLEEP	NOTES
Before	2h after							

DATE	BREAKFAST		MEDICINE	LUNCH		MEDICINE	DINNER		MEDICINE
	Before	2h after		Before	2h after		Before	2h after	

SNACK		MEDICINE	BEDTIME	NIGHT	EXERCISE	STRESS	SLEEP	NOTES
Before	2h after							

DATE	BREAKFAST		MEDICINE	LUNCH		MEDICINE	DINNER		MEDICINE
	Before	2h after		Before	2h after		Before	2h after	

SNACK		MEDICINE	BEDTIME	NIGHT	EXERCISE	STRESS	SLEEP	NOTES
Before	2h after							

DATE	BREAKFAST		MEDICINE	LUNCH		MEDICINE	DINNER		MEDICINE
	Before	2h after		Before	2h after		Before	2h after	

SNACK		MEDICINE	BEDTIME	NIGHT	EXERCISE	STRESS	SLEEP	NOTES
Before	2h after							

DATE	BREAKFAST		MEDICINE	LUNCH		MEDICINE	DINNER		MEDICINE
	Before	2h after		Before	2h after		Before	2h after	

SNACK		MEDICINE	BEDTIME	NIGHT	EXERCISE	STRESS	SLEEP	NOTES
Before	2h after							

DATE	BREAKFAST		MEDICINE	LUNCH		MEDICINE	DINNER		MEDICINE
	Before	2h after		Before	2h after		Before	2h after	

SNACK		MEDICINE	BEDTIME	NIGHT	EXERCISE	STRESS	SLEEP	NOTES
Before	2h after							

DATE	BREAKFAST		MEDICINE	LUNCH		MEDICINE	DINNER		MEDICINE
	Before	2h after		Before	2h after		Before	2h after	

SNACK		MEDICINE	BEDTIME	NIGHT	EXERCISE	STRESS	SLEEP	NOTES
Before	2h after							

DATE	BREAKFAST		MEDICINE	LUNCH		MEDICINE	DINNER		MEDICINE
	Before	2h after		Before	2h after		Before	2h after	

SNACK		MEDICINE	BEDTIME	NIGHT	EXERCISE	STRESS	SLEEP	NOTES
Before	2h after							

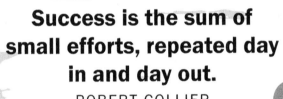

Success is the sum of small efforts, repeated day in and day out.

ROBERT COLLIER

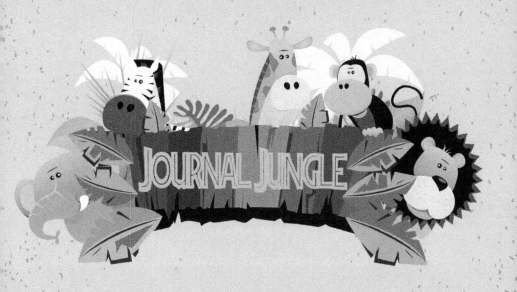

VISIT US ONLINE TO CHECK OUT OUR FULL
COLLECTION OF JOURNALS, WORKBOOKS,
COLORING BOOKS, ACTIVITY BOOKS & MORE!!

WWW.JOURNALJUNGLE.COM

Made in the USA
Monee, IL
18 February 2021